Causesofcancerandit'sprevention

unhealthypracticeswecarryoutinourday-to-daylivesthatcancausecancer.

DrAshley.G.Silvia

Copyright2023.

Pleasenotethatthisisageneraloutlineandyoumayneedtocustomizeitbasedonyourspecificrequirementsorthetargetaudience.Itisalwaysrecommendedtoconsultreliablesourcesandmedicalprofessionalsforaccurateandup-to-dateinformationoncancercausesandpreventioninourday-to-daylives.

troduction

hereoncewasawomannamedMelaniewholivedinthebusycityofMetropolis.Beingadrivenandaspira
onalperson,Melaniewasconstantlypushingherselftodobetter.Shewasanenthusiasticsmoker,thou
h,whichwasonebadhabitshefounddifficulttobreak.

ithoutrealizingthepossibleriskstoherhealth,Melaniehadbeenasmokerformanyyears.Unbeknown
toher,herhabitwasgraduallyincreasingherchanceofcancer.Luckilyforher,fatehadotherideas.

chroniccoughthatMelaniehaddevelopedwasspottedonedaybyherclosefriendLisa,whoalsohappe
stobeanurse.LisapushedMelanietogetathoroughmedicalcheckupbecauseshewasworriedabouth
rpal.

elanie,whohadpreviouslydismissedherfriend'sconcerns,finallyconsentedtoseeawell-
nownoncologistinthecity.

heoncologistevaluatedMelanie'sgeneralhealthduringhervisitbyrunningseveraltestsandscreening
Heramazementwascompoundedbytheresults,whichshowedpossibleprecancerouscellsandearly
gnsoflungdamage.Melanie'ssmokinghabitmayhavecontributedtothedevelopmentoflungcancer,t
edoctornoted,ifithadgoneunnoticedanduntreated.

elaniewashorrifiedandstartledbythenews,andsherecognizedtheseriousnessofherterriblebehavi
r.Shedecidedtogiveupsmokingforgood,andtohelpherwiththis,shesoughtexpertassistance.Melani
startedherquesttostopsmokingwiththehelpofherlovedones,friends,andafocusedprogram.

Melaniesetoutonaquesttoovercomeheraddiction.

Melanie'shealthprogressivelygotbetterasthemonthspassed.Sheexperiencedareductioninherchro
niccoughandanincreaseinherenergylevels.Shestartedtopromotehealthylivingandtookanactivepa
incampaignstoraiseawarenessoftherisksassociatedwithsmoking.

Melanie'sexperienceservesasapotentreminderofthevalueofpreventionandearlydetection.Shewa
abletopreventtheterribleoutcomesthatsmokingcouldhavebroughtaboutbyquicklyaddressingherb
dhabitandgettingmedicalattention.Numerouspeopleweremotivatedbyherstorytotakechargeofthe
healthandmakelife-improvingdecisions.

Melaniebecameasymboloftenacityandwillpowerafterthatday,servingasaconstantremindertoever
onethatit'snevertoolatetomakeachangeinyourlifeandgiveyourhealthpriority.

Chapterone:Definitionandtypesofcancer

Theuncheckedgrowthanddisseminationofaberrantcellswithinthebodyisthehallmarkofthecomplexd
seaseknownascancer.Theseaberrantcellsalsoreferredtoascancercells,caninvadeandkillnearbyti
ssuesandorgans.Differenttypesofcancerexist,andtheyarecategorizedaccordingtotheparticularcell
ortissuesfromwhichtheyoriginate.Skin,lung,prostate,colorectal,andbreastcancersareafewcomm
oncancertypes.Itiscrucialtorememberthateverytypeofcancerhasnumeroussubtypesandvariations,
eachwithspecialtraitsandmethodsoftreatment.

Itiscrucialtocomprehendthecausesandpreventativemeasuresofcancer
formultiplereasons:

1.Earlydetectionandprevention:Peoplecanlowertheirriskofcancerbymakingeducatedlifestyledecisi
onsandtakingpreventiveactionsafterlearningaboutthedisease'scauses.Thisentailsforminghealthfu
routineslikeeatingabalanceddiet,workingoutfrequently,abstainingfromtobaccoandexcessivealcoh
oluse,andshieldingoneselffromdangerousenvironmentalelementslikeUVrays.

2.Bettertreatmentresults:Targetedtherapiesandinterventionscanbedevelopedasaresultofabetteru
nderstandingofthecausesofcancer.Forinstance,ifacertaingeneticmutationisconnectedtoaparticula
kindofcancer,scientistscanconcentrateoncreatingmedicationsthatspecificallytargetthatmutation,r
esultinginmoreefficientandindividualizedtreatmentchoices.

3.Publichealthinitiatives:Understandingthecausesofcanceraidspolicymakersandpublichealthgrou
psincreatingplanstolessenthefinancialburdenthatcancerplacesonsociety.Thisentailsputtingcancer
screeningprogramsintoaction,raisingawarenessthroughcampaigns,andarguinginfavoroflawsthate
ncouragecancerpreventionandearlydetection.

4.Empoweringpeople:Knowingthecausesofcancerenablespeopletotakechargeoftheirhealthandm
akewisedecisions.Earlydetectionandimprovedtreatmentoutcomescanresultfrompeople'sabilitytoi
dentifypotentialriskfactorsandseekappropriatemedicaladvice.

5.Reducingrisk:Peoplecanrecognizeandalterriskfactorsintheirsurroundingsandwayoflifebylearnin
gaboutthecausesofcancer.Peoplecanlessentheirchanceofgettingcancerbymakingeducateddecisi
ons,suchasmaintainingahealthydiet,exercisingfrequently,abstainingfromtobaccoandexcessivealc
oholuse,andshieldingthemselvesfromcarcinogens.

6.Innovationandresearchadvancementsarefueledbyourgrowingunderstandingofthecausesofcanc
er.Itfacilitatesthediscoveryofnoveltreatmentmodalities,potentialpreventivemeasures,andnewriskf
actorsbyresearchers.Thisinformationadvancesongoinginitiativestoenhancecancerdetection,prev
ention,andcare.

Finally,itshouldbenotedthatresearchadvancements,publichealthinitiatives,earlydetection,targeted
interventions,riskreduction,andpersonalempowermentalldependonanunderstandingofthecauses
andpreventionofcancer.Bylearningmoreaboutthesetopics,wecanallworktogethertoimprovegenera
lhealthoutcomesandlessentheimpactofcancer.

Understandingcancercauses

Scientificresearch,epidemiologicalstudies,andindividualriskassessmentareallintegralcomponents
ofacomprehensiveapproachtounderstandingcancercauses.Tolearnmoreaboutthecausesofcancer
followtheseimportantsteps:

.Beknowledgeable:Stayabreastofthemostrecentfindingsanddataregardingthecausesofcancer.A
uthenticresourceslikerespectablemedicaljournals,cancerresearchorganizations,andgovernmenth
ealthagenciescanofferinsightfulinformationaboutthestateofourknowledgeregardingthecauseofcan
ceratthemoment.

2:Investigateriskfactors:Listandresearchtheestablishedriskfactorsconnectedtovariouscancertype
s.Predispositiontocancercanbeinherited,exposuretocarcinogens(tobaccosmokeorspecificchemic
als),lifestyledecisions(dietandexercise),infections,hormonalchanges,andenvironmentalfactorsca
nallberiskfactors.
3.Examineepidemiologicalresearch:Studiesthatlookattrendsandconnectionsbetweencancerincid
enceandriskfactorsarecalledepidemiologicalresearch.Thisresearchcanofferimportantinformation
abouttheconnectionbetweenparticularexposuresorlifestylechoicesandtheonsetofcancer.Findingp
robablecausesandriskfactorscanbeaidedbyreadingthroughandcomprehendingthesestudies.

4.Speakwithmedicalexperts:Talktomedicalexperts,suchasoncologists,geneticcounselors,orprima
rycarephysicians,aboutyourworriesandinquiriesregardingthecausesofcancer.Takingintoaccounty
ouruniqueriskfactors,familyhistory,andmedicalhistory,theycanoffertailoredadvice.

5.Evaluatepersonalrisk:Takeintoaccountyourlifestylechoices,familyhistory,andexposuretopossib
ecarcinogenswhenassessingyourcancerriskfactors.Tomakewisechoicesaboutscreeningsandpre
entativemeasures,youcanusethisinformationtobetterunderstandyourriskprofile.

6.Takepartinstudies:Takeintoconsiderationtakingpartinclinicaltrialsorresearchprojectsthatexamin
ethecausesofcancer.Inadditiontopossiblygainingaccesstothemostrecentdevelopmentsincancerp
eventionandtreatment,youcanfurtheryourunderstandingofthecausesofcancerbymakingcontributio
nstoscience.

Recallthattherearenumerouscontributingvariablestocancer,makingitacomplicateddiseasewhosep
recisecauseisfrequentlyunknown.Ontheotherhand,youcanimproveyourcomprehensionbyremaini
nginformed,evaluatingyourownrisk,andtakingpreventativemeasures.

eneticfactors

theemergenceofcancer,geneticfactorsareveryimportant.Anindividual'svulnerabilitytosomeforms
fcancermaybeincreasedbyspecificinheritedgenemutations.Cancerriskcanbeconsiderablyraised
ythesemutations,whichcanbeinheritedfromparentstotheiroffspring.Ahigherriskofbreastandovaria
cancerislinkedtocertaingeneticmutations,suchasthoseinBRCA1andBRCA2.Therearealsoknown
eneticsyndromesthatraisetheriskofdevelopingmorethanonetypeofcancer,includingLi-
raumenisyndromeandLynchsyndrome.Itiscrucialtorememberthatotherenvironmentalandlifestyle
ctorsalsoplayapartinthedevelopmentofcancer,eventhoughgeneticfactorscanplayasignificantrole
itsdevelopment.Genetictestingandroutinescreeningscanaidpeopleinrecognizingtheirriskandado
tingthenecessaryprecautions.

nvironmentalfactors

ancerdevelopmentcanalsobestronglyinfluencedbyenvironmentalfactors.Thechanceofgettingdiff
rentkindsofcancercanrisewhenexposedtospecificenvironmentalfactorsandsubstances.Typicale
vironmentalvariableslinkedtocancerinclude:

.Carcinogens:Theriskofacquiringcancercanberaisedbyexposuretosubstancesknowntocausecan
er,includingasbestos,tobaccosmoke,somechemicals,andradiation.

.Airandwaterpollution:Peoplewholiveinareaswithpoorairqualityorcontaminatedwatersourcesmay
eexposedtodangerouschemicalsthatmayhastentheonsetofcancer.

.Hazardsassociatedwiththeworkplace:Thereisachancethatapersonworkinginajobthatexposesth
mtochemicals,radiation,orasbestoswillgetcancerfromtheirjob.

.Lifestyledecisions:Smoking,bingedrinking,eatingpoorly,andnotgettingenoughexercisereallunh
althylifestylechoicesthatcandramaticallyraiseone'sriskofcancer.

kincancerriskcanbeelevatedbyprolongedexposuretoultraviolet(UV)radiation,whichcanbederived
omthesunortanningbeds.

educedriskofcancer-
latedtoenvironmentalfactorscanbeachievedbyadoptingahealthylifestyle,minimizingexposuretok
owncarcinogens,andadheringtoadvisedsafetyguidelines.Identificationandtreatmentofcancerata
earlystagealsodependonroutinescreeningsandearlydetection.

Lifestylefactors

Theonsetofcancermaybesignificantlyinfluencedbylifestylechoices.Aperson'sriskofgettingacertai
kindofcancercanberaisedbyspecificdecisionsandactions.Ahigherriskofcancerislinkedtothefollowi
glifestylefactors:

1.Useoftobaccoproducts:Smokingtobaccoproducts,suchascigarettes,cigars,andpipes,isamajorc
useofcancerinthemouth,throat,bladder,andlungs.Itcanalsobedetrimentaltobearoundsecondhand
moke.

2.Dietandnutrition:Consumingadiethighinprocessedfoods,redandprocessedmeats,unhealthyfats
andlowinfruits,vegetables,andwholegrainscanraiseyourriskofdevelopingcertaincancers,includin
colorectalcancer.Dietcanaffectobesity,whichisalsoconnectedtoanelevateddangerofvariouscance
kinds.

3.Inactivity:Thereisalinkbetweenirregularphysicalactivityandahigherchanceofdevelopingsomeca
cers,suchasendometrial,breast,andcoloncancer.Regularexercisecanhelplowertherisk.

4.Alcoholintake:Itiswellrecognizedthatconsumingexcessiveamountsofalcoholincreasestheriskof
evelopingliver,breast,colorectal,andoralcancers.Itisadvisedtominimizeorstayawayfromalcoholco
mpletely.

5.Sunexposure:ExcessiveexposuretoUVradiationfromtanningbedsorthesuncanraisetheriskofme
anomaandotherskincancers.Usingsunscreenandshieldingtheskinfromprolongedsunexposurear
crucialpreventativesteps.

Peoplecanlowertheirriskofdevelopingcancerbyleadingahealthylifestyle,whichincludesabstaining
omtobaccouse,eatingabalanceddiet,exercisingfrequently,consumingnomorealcoholthannecessa
ry,andusingsunscreenexcessively.Identificationandtreatmentofcanceratanearlystagealsodepen
onroutinescreeningsandearlydetection.

Occupationalfactors

Somecancersmaydevelopasaresultoffactorsrelatedtotheworkplace.Occupationallyrelatedcancer scanbemorelikelytooccurwhenworkersareexposedtospecificsubstancesandhazards.Followingare afewtypicalwork-relatedriskfactorsforcancer:

1.Asbestos:Mesothelioma,lungcancer,andotherrespiratorymalignanciescanresultfromexposureto asbestosfibersbyworkersinindustrieslikeshipbuilding,construction,andinsulationmanufacturing.

2.Chemicals:Workersinindustriesincludingmanufacturing,agriculture,andchemicalproductionarea ahigherriskofdevelopinglung,bladder,andleukemiacancersduetoexposuretocertainchemicalslike benzene,formaldehyde,arsenic,andcertainsolvents.

3.Radiation:Employeesworkinginnuclearpower,radiology,andsomehealthcareenvironmentsmayb esubjectedtoionizingradiation,whichraisestheriskofcancer,especiallythyroidandleukemia.

4.Heavymetals:Cancersofthekidney,lung,andotherorganscanariseasaresultofexposuretoheavym etalssuchascadmium,lead,andchromiuminthemining,battery,andmetalworkingindustries.

5.Shiftwork:Workinglongnightshasbeenlinkedtoahigherriskofcolorectalandbreastcancer,presuma blyasaresultofmelatoninproductionandcircadianrhythmdisruptions.

Employersshouldplaceahighpriorityonworkplacesafety,supplyappropriatesafetygear,andputpolici esinplacetoreduceexposuretocarcinogens.Appropriatetraining,followingsafetyregulations,androu tineobservationcanaidinloweringtheriskofcancerslinkedtotheworkplace.

InfectiousAgents
Thedevelopmentofcancerhasbeenlinkedtospecificinfectiousagentsasriskfactors.Thesesubstance
shavethepotentialtocausecancerdirectlyortoraisetheriskofdevelopingit.Togiveafewinstances:
1.ThefirstisthehumanpapillomavirusorHPV.Thissexuallytransmittedinfectioncancausecancersoft
hecervical,anal,andotherregions,aswellascertaincancersoftheheadandneck.

2.TheriskoflivercancercanbeelevatedbyapersistentinfectionwitheitherthehepatitisBorCvirus.

3.Thehumanimmunodeficiencyvirus(HIV)increasestheriskofdevelopingcertaincancers,includingn
on-Hodgkinlymphoma,cervicalcancer,andKaposisarcoma.

4.Epstein-
Barrvirus(EBV):BRCA,nasopharyngealcarcinoma,Burkittlymphoma,andcertaincasesofHodgkinly
mphomaareamongthecancerslinkedtoEBV.

5.AdultT-cellleukemia/lymphomaisassociatedwithhumanT-celllymphotropicvirustype1(HTLV-1).

Noteveryonewhocontractsoneoftheseinfectiousagentswillgoontogetcancer,itisimportanttoremem
ber.Ontheotherhand,exposuretotheseagentscanraisetherisk;avoidanceofsharedneedlesandsafe
sexualpractices,forexample,canhelplowertheriskofcancerslinkedtotheseagents.Managingandtrea
tingtheseinfectionsandassociatedcancersalsodependsheavilyonroutinescreeningsandearlydetec
tion.

Lifestylefactors

Numerouslifestylefactorshavebeenconnectedtoahigherriskofcancer.Amongthemare:

1.Tobaccouse:Theriskofdevelopinglung,mouth,throat,esophageal,andbladdercancersisincrease
dbysmokingcigarettes,cigars,orpipesaswellasbyusingsmokelesstobaccoproducts.

2.Unhealthydiet:Consumingadiethighinprocessedfoods,redandprocessedmeats,sugarybeverage
s,andlowinfruits,vegetables,andwholegrainshasbeenlinkedtoanincreasedriskofcancer,especially
colorectalcancer.

3.Physicalinactivity:Livingasedentarylifestylewithlittletonoexercisehasbeenassociatedwithahigher
riskofdevelopingcertaincancers,includingbreastandcoloncancer.

4.Overindulgenceinalcohol:Studieshaveindicatedthatfrequentandheavyalcoholuseraisestheriskof
severalcancers,includingthoseoftheliver,mouth,throat,esophagus,breast,andcolon.

5.Exposuretohazardouschemicals:Environmentalexposuretopesticidesandpollutants,aswellasoc
cupationalexposuretochemicalslikeformaldehyde,benzene,andasbestos,canraisetheriskofcancer

It'scrucialtorememberthatalthoughleadingtheselifestylechoicescanraiseyourchanceofdeveloping
cancer,theydonotensureitwill.Inaddition,theriskofdevelopingcancerisinfluencedbyadditionalvariab
leslikehereditandfamilyhistory.Fortailoredcounselanddirectiononcancerprevention,itisalwaysadv
isabletospeakwithahealthcareprovider.

Tobaccoandsmokinguse

Ahigherriskofcanceriscloselyassociatedwithtobaccouse,especiallysmoking.Aconsiderableportion
ofcancercasesarecausedbysmokingtobacco,whichistheworld'slargestpreventablecauseofdeath.
Concerningtobaccouseandcancer,thefollowingareimportantpoints:

Lungcancer:Becausesmokingcauseslungcancerinapproximately85%ofcases,itisthemaincauseof
ungcancer.Toxinsandcarcinogensfoundintobaccosmokedamagelungtissueandmaycausethegro
wthofcanceroustumorsbydamaginglungcells.

2.Othercancertypes:Usingtobaccoalsoraisesyourriskofdevelopingmouth,throat,esophageal,blad
er,kidney,pancreatic,cervical,andcolorectalcancers,amongothers.Additionally,itmayhelptothegro
wthofcancersinotherbodyregions.

3.Secondhandsmoke:Smokefromburningtobaccoproductsortheexhaledbysmokerscanraisetheris
kofcancerinnonsmokers.Manyofthesamedangeroussubstancesfoundinsmokethatisinhaleddirect
yarealsopresentinsecondhandsmoke.

4.Givingupsmoking:Givingupsmokingdramaticallylowersyourriskofacquiringcancer.Overtime,the
ecanbehealthbenefitsandadecreasedriskofcancerevenforlong-
termsmokerswhogiveup.Itisnevertoolatetostartlivingahealthierlifestyleandgiveupsmoking.

5.Othertobaccoproducts:Althoughsmokingcigarettesisthemostwell-
knowntobaccousemethod,thereareothermethodsaswell,includingcigars,pipes,andsmokelesstoba
ccoproducts(likesnufforchewingtobacco),whichalsoraisetheriskofcancer.Thesegoodsaremadewi
hdangerousingredientsthatcandamagecellsandleadto
Cancer.

Recognizingthedangersoftobaccouseandsmoking,aswellasseekingassistanceandresourcestohe
pyoustop,isessentialifyousmoke.Healthcareprovidersandorganizationsthatspecializeinsmokingce
ssationcanoffertailoredadviceandsupportforquitting,whichcanlowertheriskofcancer.

DietandNutrition

Overallhealthandthepreventionofcanceraresignificantlyinfluencedbydietandnutrition.Thefollowing
aresomeimportantdetailsaboutdietandcancerrisk:

.Plant-
baseddiet:Researchhaslinkedadiethighinfruits,vegetables,wholegrains,andlegumestoadecrease
riskofdevelopingseveralcancers.Thesefoodsarerichinantioxidants,fiber,vitamins,andmineralstha
helppreventcellulardamageandlowertheriskofcancer.

.ReduceYourIntakeofProcessedandRedMeats:Studieshaveshownaconnectionbetweenahigherr
skofcolorectalcancerandhigherconsumptionofprocessedmeats(likebacon,sausages,anddelimeat
)andredmeats(likebuffalo,hog,andlamb).Leanproteinsourceslikefish,poultry,andplant-
basedproteinsarepreferabletothesemeatswhenitcomestoconsumingyourprotein.

.Lessenyourintakeofprocessedfoodsandsugar-
filledbeverages:Consumingalotoftheseitemshasbeenlinkedtoanincreasedriskofobesity,whichrais
stheriskofdevelopingmanycancers.Sugar-
filleddrinksshouldbeavoidedasmuchaspossible;instead,sticktowholefoods,water,anddrinkswithou
addedsugar.

.Keepyourweightwithinahealthyrange:Obesityandoverweightraisetheriskofcolorectal,kidney,pan
reatic,breast,andothercancers.Reducingtheriskofcancerandmaintainingahealthyweightcanbeac
ievedbycombiningabalanceddietwithregularexercise.

.Remainhydrated:Eatingahealthydietandstayinghydratedisimportantforcancerpreventionaswella
overallhealth.Itfacilitatestheremovaloftoxinsfromthebodyandkeepsphysiologicalprocessesfuncti
ningproperly.

Whileahealthydietcanreducetheriskofcancer,preventionisnotguaranteedbyit,itisimportanttoreme
berthis.Cancerriskisalsoinfluencedbyadditionalvariableslikegenetics,wayoflife,andexposuretoth
environment.Aregistereddietitianorotherhealthcareprofessionalshouldbeconsultedforspecificrec
mmendationsregardingnutritionanddietincancerprevention.

PhysicalActivityandExercise
Exerciseandphysicalactivityhavebeendemonstratedtopositivelyaffecttheriskofsomecancertypes.
Frequentexercisehelpsreducetheriskofgettingcancer,includinglung,endometrial,breast,andcolon
ancer.Thefollowingaresomeimportantdetailsaboutphysicalactivityandcancer:

1.Lowerriskofcancer:Studieshavelinkedregularphysicalactivitytoadecreasedriskofsomecancerty
es.Exerciseisthoughttolowerinflammation,boostthebody'scapacitytorepairDNAdamage,helpregu
atehormonelevels,andimproveimmunefunction,allofwhichmaylowertheriskofdevelopingcancer.

2.Breastcancer:Researchindicatesthatwomenwhoregularlyworkout,evenifit'sjustmoderatelyinter
seaerobicwalkingorrunning,arelesslikelytodevelopbreastcancer.Exercisehasthepotentialtolower
strogenlevels,whichmaycontributetothedevelopmentofbreastcancer.

3.Coloncancer:Studieshaveshownacorrelationbetweenaregularexerciseregimenandalowerrisko
coloncancer.Exercisehasthepotentialtolowertheriskofcoloncancerbyenhancingbowelfunction,red
ucinginflammationinthecolon,andspeedingupthepassageoffoodthroughthedigestivesystem.

4.Endometrialcancer:Studieshavelinkedphysicalactivitytoalowerriskofthistypeofcancer.Exercise
anhelpyoukeepahealthyweight,controlyourhormonelevels,andenhanceinsulinsensitivity,allofwhi
hcouldbelinkedtoadecreasedriskofendometrialcancer.

5.Lungcancer:Althoughregularphysicalactivityhasbeendemonstratedtohaveaprotectiveeffect,esp
eciallyinnon-
smokers,smokingremainstheprimaryriskfactorforlungcancer.Engaginginphysicalactivityhasthepo
entialtomitigatetheriskoflungcancerbyaugmentingimmunesystemperformance,decreasinginflam
mation,andimprovinglungfunction.

Itissignificanttorememberthattheprecisequantityandqualityofphysicalactivityneededtolowertheris
ofcancermaydifferbasedonpersonalfactorslikeage,generalhealth,andleveloffitness.Aimforatleast
50minutesofmoderate-intenseaerobicactivityor75minutesofvigorous-
intenseaerobicactivityeachweek,anddostrengthtrainingexercisesatleasttwiceaweek.Asusual,it'sb
esttospeakwithamedicalexpert,Beforebeginninganynewexerciseroutine.

Alcoholconsumption

Ahigherriskofdevelopingsomeformsofcancerhasbeenassociatedwithalcoholconsumption.Ithasbe
endemonstratedbyresearchthatfrequentandexcessivealcoholusecanincreasetheriskofdeveloping
manycancers,suchasthoseoftheliver,mouth,throat,esophagus,breast,andcolon.Thereisapositivec
orrelationbetweenalcoholconsumptionandcancerrisk.Remarkably,therecanstillbesomeriskassoci
atedwithmoderatealcoholconsumption.Itisrecommendedtorestrictalcoholconsumptionorevencon
sidergivingitupcompletelytolowertheriskofcancer.Forspecificcounselanddirection,itisalwaysadvis
edtospeakwithahealthcareprofessional.

ObesityandBodyweight
Excessbodyweightandobesityareimportantriskfactorsformanycancertypes.Studieshaveindicatedt
hatbeingobeseoroverweightraisestheriskofdevelopingmultiplecancers,suchasliver,kidney,pancre
atic,breast,colorectal,andendometrialcancers.Althoughthepreciseprocessesbywhichobesityleads
tothedevelopmentofcancerarenotentirelyunderstood,itisthoughtthatobesitycancauseinsulinresist
ance,hormonalimbalances,andchronicinflammation,allofwhichcanencouragethegrowthofcancerc
ells.Abalanceddietandregularexercisesareessentialformaintainingahealthybodyweight,whichlower
stheriskofcancerandenhancesgeneralhealth.Seekingadvicefromahealthcareproviderisalwaysadv
isedforrecommendationsandindividualizedadvice.
SunExposureandUVRadiation
OneknownriskfactorforskincancerisexposuretoultravioJet(UV)lightandthesun.Skincancercanarise
asaresultofDNAdamagetoskincellscausedbyprolonged,unprotectedexposuretoUVradiationfromth
esun.BothartificialUVradiationsources,liketanningbeds,andnaturalsunlightfallunderthiscategory.B
asalcellcarcinomaandsquamouscellcarcinomaarethetwoprimaryformsofskincancerlinkedtosunex
posure;thesetwotypesofcancerareoftenlessaggressive.Yet,melanoma,amoreseriouskindofskinca
ncer,canalsobemorelikelytodevelopasaresultofprolongedsunexposure.

It'scriticaltoexercisecautionwhenexposedtothesuntolowertheriskofskincancer.Thisentailsconsiste
ntlyusinghigh-
SPFsunscreen,lookingforshadeduringthehottestpartsoftheday,anddressingprotectivelywithhatsa
ndlong-
sleevedshirts.TanningbedsshouldalsobecompletelyavoidedbecausetheyreleasedangerousUVray
s.Thediagnosisandtreatmentofskincancerdependheavilyonroutineskinexamsandearlydetection.Iti
sadvisedtoseekindividualizedadviceandguidancefromadermatologistorhealthcareprofessionalify
ouhaveconcernsregardingsunexposureanditscorrelationwithcancer.

Environmentalexposures(e.gAirpollution,chemicals)
Cancerdevelopmentmaybeinfluencedbypollutionandenvironmentalexposures.Sincetheyhavethe
potentialtocausecancer,someenvironmentalpollutantsandsubstanceshavebeenclassifiedascarci
ogens.Someoftheseincludeexposuretoradiation,industrialemissions,waterandsoilcontaminants,a
ndairpollutantslikeparticulatematterandspecificchemicals.

Inhalingcontaminatedair,consumingcontaminatedfoodorwater,orcomingintodirectcontactwithhaz
ardousmaterialsatworkarejustafewwaysthatpeoplecanbecomeexposedtothesecarcinogens.Thep
articularcancersthatareassociatedwithenvironmentalexposuresdifferbasedonthetypeofexposurea
ndatwhatlevel.

Nottomentionthatindividualsusceptibilityandothervariables,likegeneticsandlifestylechoices,alsop
ayapartincancerrisk,eventhoughenvironmentalexposuresandpollutioncanincreasechances.Over
allhealthcanbeimprovedandtheriskofcancercanbereducedbyminimizingexposuretoenvironmenta
pollutantsandexercisinggoodenvironmentalstewardship.Toreduceexposure,it'sagoodideatokeep
upwithpotentialenvironmentalhazardsandabidebyrulesandregulationsestablishedbyyourlocalauth
orities.Speakingwithenvironmentalspecialistsandmedicalprofessionalscanhelpyoureducetherisks
thatcomewithbeingexposedtotheenvironment.

Cancerpreventionstrategiesindailylife
Reducingtheriskofcancercanbeaccomplishedbyimplementingcancerpreventionstrategiesintoeve
ydaylife.Followingareafewsuggestionssupportedbyevidence:

Tokeepyourweightincheck,eatabalanceddietfulloffruits,vegetables,wholegrains,andleanmeats.C
onsumingprocessedfoods,sugar-filledbeverages,andhigh-
caloriesnacksshouldbeminimized.Forthemanagementofweight,regularphysicalactivityisalsocruci
al.

2.Steerclearoftobacco:Manycancersarelargelycausedbysmokingandtobaccouse.Avoidbeingarou
ndsecondhandsmokeandgethelpifyousmoketostop.

3.Moderatealcoholintake:Excessivealcoholintakehasbeenassociatedwithahigherriskofseveralca
cers.It'sbesttorestrictalcoholconsumptionorthinkaboutgivingitupcompletely.

4.Protectfromthesun:Skincancerriskisincreasedbyexposuretoultraviolet(UV)radiationfromthesun
ortanningbeds.Usehigh-
SPFsunscreen,coverupwithprotectiveclothes,andseekoutshadeduringthehottestpartsofthedaytop
rotectyourskin.

5.Obtainavaccination:HepatitisBandthehumanpapillomavirus(HPV)canraiseyourriskofcontracting
certaincancers.Therearevaccinationsavailabletoguardagainsttheseinfections.

6.Havesafesexualinteractions:Avoidsexuallytransmittedinfections(STIs),suchasHPV,whichcanca
usecervicalandothercancers.Instead,adoptsafesexualbehaviors.

7.Maintainyourphysicalfitness:Getatleast150minutesaweekofmoderate-to-
ntenseexercise,suchascycling,jogging,orbriskwalking.Inadditiontoloweringtheriskofcertaincancer
s,physicalactivityhelpspeoplemaintainahealthyweight.

8.Screeningandearlydetection:Forcancerslikebreast,cervical,colorectal,andprostatecancer,adher
etorecommendedscreeningguidelines.Treatmentresultscanbeconsiderablyenhancedbyearlydete
ction.

Theytheycangreatlyreducetheriskofdevelopingcancer,keepinmindthatthesetacticsarenot100%
effective.Seekingguidancefromahealthcareprofessionalanddiscussinganyparticularconcernsisal
waysrecommendedsuchasafamilyhistoryofcancer.

Tobaccocontrolandsmokingcessation
Topreventcancer,itisimperativetocontroltobaccouseandquitsmoking.Cancersofthemouth,throat,e
sophagus,bladder,andlungsareamongthemanycancersthatareprimarilybroughtonbytobaccouse.
Thechanceofgettingthesecancerscanbegreatlydecreasedbygivingupsmokingandabstainingfroma
lltobaccouse.

Reducedsmokingratesandthepreventionofcancerhavebeenachievedthroughtheuseoftobaccocon
rolmeasureslikeraisingtaxesontobaccoproducts,enactingsmoke-
freelaws,andlaunchingpublicawarenesscampaigns.Theobjectivesoftheseinitiativesaretodetertob
accouse,shieldnonsmokersfromsecondhandsmoke,andencouragetheestablishmentofsmoke-
freespaces.

Toassistpeopleinquittingsmoking,resources,andprogramsarealsocrucial.Counseling,supportgrou
ps,medication,andnicotinereplacementtherapyaresomeoftheprogramsthatmaybeincluded.Benefi
sofquittingsmokingincludealowerriskofcanceraswellasshort-andlong-termhealthbenefits.

Inadditiontogovernmentsandorganizationscontinuingtoimplementtobaccocontrolmeasures,smok
ersmustseekoutresourcesandsupporttostop.Topreventcancerandimprovegeneralhealth,itcanbev
eryhelpfultospeakwithmedicalprofessionalsandmakeuseoftheresourcesavailabletohelpquitsmoki
ng.

HealthyEatingHabits

Iswell-
recognizedthatadoptingahealthydietcansignificantlyreducetheriskofdevelopingcancer.Adietrichin
nutrientsandwell-
balancedcanhelplowertheriskofdevelopingsomeformsofcancer.Thefollowingaresomeimportantthi
ngstothinkabout:

.Consumearangeoffruitsandvegetables:Thesefoodsarehighinantioxidants,vitamins,andminerals
hatcanhelppreventcancer.Whenarrangingyourplate,trytousearangeofcolorsforthefruitsandveget
ablesonit.

.Optforwholegrains:Richinfiberandothervitalnutrients,wholegrainsincludequinoa,brownrice,and
wholewheatbread.Theycansupplylong-lastingenergyandhelpreducetheriskofcolorectalcancer.

.Reduceyourintakeofredandprocessedmeats:Redmeatslikebeefandpig,aswellasprocessedmeat
likehotdogsandbacon,havebeenrelatedtoanincreasedriskofcolorectalcanceramongothercancers
Reducingintakeandchoosingleanproteinsourcessuchasfish,poultry,andplant-
basedproteinsisthebestcourseofaction.

.Cutbackonsugar-
lledfoodsandbeverages:Consumingalotofsugarhasbeenlinkedtoobesity,whichraisestheriskofdev
lopingseveralcancers.Restricttheamountofsugarysnacks,sweets,anddrinksyouconsume.

.Selecthealthyfats:Includefoodslikeavocados,nuts,seeds,andoliveoilinyourdietassourcesofhealt
yfats.Inadditiontoofferingvitalnutrients,thesefatshaveanti-inflammatoryproperties.

.Remainhydrated:Toensureoptimalhydrationandpromotegeneralhealth,siponlotsofwaterthrough
uttheday.

ecallthatalthoughadoptinggoodeatingpracticescanreducetheriskofcancer,doingsoisonlyonepart
fanall-
ncompassingstrategyforthedisease'sprevention.It'salsocriticaltofollowmedicalprofessionals'reco
mendationsregardingcancerscreenings,abstainfromtobaccoandexcessivealcoholuse,andpartici
ateinregularphysicalactivity.

Importanceofregularphysicalactivity
Oneimportantfactorinthepreventionofsomecancersisregularphysicalactivity.Physicalactivityisstro
nglylinkedtoalowerriskofdevelopingdifferenttypesofcancer,accordingtonumerousstudies.

Numerousmechanismsexistthatexplainwhyregularexercisecanhelppreventcancer.Inthefirstplace
physicalactivitypromotesahealthybodyweight,andobesityisrecognizedtobeariskfactorforseveralca
ncers,includingkidney,pancreatic,endometrial,breast,andcolorectal.Reducingtheriskofdeveloping
thesecancerscanbeachievedthroughregularphysicalactivityandmaintainingahealthyweight.

Second,hormoneregulationinthebodycanbeaidedbyregularexercise.Anincreasedriskofbreastand
endometrialcancerhasbeenassociatedwithhighlevelsofsomehormones,suchasestrogen.Engage
mentinExercise,Frequentphysicalactivityisakeycomponentinthepreventionofsomecancers.Nume
ousstudieshaveshownastrongcorrelationbetweenphysicalactivityandalowerriskofdevelopingvario
usformsofcancer.

Thereareavarietyofexplanationsforwhyregularexercisecanhelppreventcancer.Firstofall,exercisee
ncouragesahealthyweight,andobesityhasbeenlinkedtoanumberofcancers,includingkidney,pancr
atic,endometrial,breast,andcoloncancers.Maintainingahealthyweightandengaginginregularphysi
alactivitycanhelplowerthechanceofacquiringthesecancers.

Second,consistentexercisecanhelpthebodyregulatehormones.Elevatedlevelsofsomehormones,i
cludingestrogen,havebeenlinkedtoanincreasedriskofendometrialandbreastcancer.

Additionally,immunesystemfunction,whichisvitalindetectingandeliminatingcancercells,canbeenh
ncedbyregularphysicalactivity.Physicalactivityhasbeendemonstratedtoboostimmunesystemfunc
on,loweringthechanceofcancerinitiationandadvancement.

Furthermore,exercisecanlessentheriskofcolorectalcancerandenhancedigestion.Frequentexercis
ehelpscontrolbowelmovements,minimizingtheamountoftimethatpotentiallydangerousmaterialsco
meintocontactwiththecolon.

It'scrucialtorememberthatalthoughengaginginregularphysicalactivitycandramaticallylowert.hecha
nceofacquiringsomecancers,Completepreventioncannotbeensuredbyit.Theonsetofcancerisalsoi
nfluencedbyothervariables,includinggenetics,wayoflife,andenvironmentalexposures.

Let'ssumupbysayingthatregularexerciseplaysasignificantroleinpreventingcancer.Inadditiontoboo
stingimmunity,regulatinghormonelevels,promotinghealthyweightmaintenance,andenhancingdige
stion,itcanalsolowertheriskofdevelopingspecificcancers.

Limiting Alcohol consumption

Reducing alcohol intake is a key component in cancer prevention. There is substantial evidence that drinking alcohol raises the risk of getting different kinds of cancer.

As a carcinogen, alcohol has the potential to cause cancer. Direct DNA damage can result in genetic mutations and the growth of cancerous cells. Furthermore, drinking alcohol can raise the synthesis of some hormones, like estrogen, which can accelerate the development of malignancies linked to hormones, such as ovarian and breast cancers.

The cancer types most closely linked to alcohol use include:

1. Breast cancer: Research has repeatedly demonstrated that even moderate alcohol use can raise a woman's risk of developing breast cancer. The more alcohol one consumes, the higher the risk.

2. Liver cancer: Due to its ability to induce cirrhosis and inflammation of the liver, both of which can lead to cancer, alcohol is a significant risk factor for liver cancer.

3. Colorectal cancer: Excessive alcohol use has been associated with a higher risk of colorectal cancer. When combined with other risk factors like smoking and eating poorly, the risk increases even more.

4. Esophageal, throat, and mouth cancer: Drinking alcohol increases the risk of developing these cancers. Consuming alcohol for longer periods and in larger quantities increases risk.

Limiting alcohol intake or abstaining from it completely is advised to lower the risk of cancer. Up to one standard drink for women and up to two standard drinks for men per day is considered moderate alcohol consumption, according to the World Health Organization (WHO).

It is significant to remember that a person's risk of developing cancer is influenced by a number of factors, such as lifestyle decisions, genetics, and general health. Reducing alcohol intake is just one part of a comprehensive strategy to prevent cancer, which also includes abstaining from tobacco use, eating a healthy diet, exercising frequently, and getting screenings on a regular basis as advised by medical professionals.

SunProtectionMeasures
Skincancerisprimarilycausedbyexposuretoultraviolet(UV)radiationfromthesun.Takingpreventativ
emeasurescanloweryourriskofdevelopingskincancersignificantly.Herearesomekeysunprotection
measurestothinkabout:

1.Seekshade:TominimizedirectUVrayexposure,seekshadeduringthesun'sstrongesthours,whicha
etypicallybetween10a.m.and4p.m.

2.Wearprotectiveclothing:Clothesthatcoverexposedskincanaddanextralayerofprotection.Choose
ong-sleevedshirts,longpants,andwide-brimmedhatstoprotectyourface,neck,andearsfromthesun.

3.Usesunscreen:Evenonovercastdays,protectallexposedskinwithabroad-
spectrumsunscreenwithanSPFof30orhigher.Everytwohours,ormorefrequentlyifyou'resweatingors
wimming,reapply.

4.Putonsunglasses:WearsunglassesthatcompletelyblockUVAandUVBraystoshieldyoureyesfrom
UVradiation.SeekforsunglasseswithUVprotectiononthelabel.

5.Steerclearofsunlampsandtanningbeds:TheseartificialUVradiationsourcescanbeequallyhazardo
usasthesun.Toloweryourriskofdevelopingskincancer,stayawayfromtanningbeds.

6.Recognizereflectivesurfaces:Sunexposurecanbeincreasedbyreflectivesurfacessuchaswater,sa
nd,andsnow.Whenspendingtimeclosetothesesurfaces,exerciseextracaution.

7.Doroutineskinself-
examinations:Lookforanychangesonyourskin,suchasgrowths,newmoles,oradjustmentstoalready
existingmoles.Seeanexpertinhealthcareifyounoticeanythingsuspect.

AsUVrayscanstillbeharmfulevenoncloudyorcoolerdays,keepinmindthatsunprotectionmeasuressh
ouldbeusedallyearround.Itispossibletoloweryourriskofskincancerandimprovethehealthofyourskin
bytakingthese.

AvoidingHarmfulEnvironmentalExposure
Preventingharmfulenvironmentalexposuresisacriticalcomponentinthemanagementofcancer.Ever
thoughthereisnowaytopreventeverycancer,peoplecanlowertheirriskbylimitingtheirexposuretoenv
ronmentalfactorsthatareknowntoraisetheriskofthedisease.

Avoidingsecondhandandtobaccosmokeisacrucialfirststep.Lung,throat,andbladdercancerarejusta
ewofthecancersthatsmokingisknowntocause.Peoplecandrasticallylowertheirriskofacquiringthese
cancersbygivingupsmokingandlimitingtheirexposuretosecondhandsmoke.

ReducingtheamountoftimespentinthesunandtanningbedsisanothercrucialprecautionagainstUVra
diation.TheprimaryriskfactorformelanomaandskincancerisexcessiveUVradiationexposure.Tored

eyourexposuretoUVrays,it'sagoodideatofindshade,wearprotectiveclothes,andapplysunscreenwi
hahighsunprotectionfactor.

Theriskofcancercanalsobedecreasedbylimitingexposuretospecificchemicalsandenvironmentalpol
utants.Avoidingorreducingexposuretohazardouschemicalspresentinpesticides,householdcleanin
gproducts,andindustrialsettingsisalsopartofthis.Asbestosislinkedtolungcancerandmesothelioma.

Maintainingahealthylifestylecanalsohelppreventcancer.Thatmeansconsuminglessprocessedandr
edmeatandstickingtoabalanceddiethighinfruits,vegetables,andwholegrains.Additionallycrucialtolo
weringtheriskofcancerareregularphysicalactivity,keepingahealthyweight,andminimizingalcoholus
e.

Notethateachpersonmaybemoreorlesssusceptibletoenvironmentalfactors,andthatwemaynotbeab
etocontrolallexposures.Nevertheless,peoplecanhelplowertheirchanceofacquiringcancerbybeing
awareofpossiblerisksandtakingproactivemeasurestolimitexposuretodangerousenvironmentalfact
ors.Inordertoidentifyandtreatanypotentialcancerousconditionsearlyon,routinecheck-
upsandscreeningsarecrucial.

Vaccinations(e.g,HPV,HepatitisB)

Certaincancers,suchasthoselinkedtoHPVandlivercancerlinkedtoHepatitisB,canbepreventedinlarg
epartbyvaccination.

Thebulkofcervical,anal,vaginal,vulvar,andoropharyngealcancersarecausedbyinfectionswithHPVt
ypesthatcanbepreventedwiththeHumanPapillomavirus(HPV)vaccine.Peoplecangreatlylowertheir
chanceofacquiringthesekindsofcancersbygettingtheHPVvaccine.Itisusuallyadministeredduringad
olescenceorearlyadulthoodandisadvisedforbothmalesandfemales.

AviralinfectioncalledhepatitisBcancausechronicliverdiseaseand,inrarecircumstances,evenliverca
ncer.OnesafeandefficientmethodofpreventingHepatitisBinfectionandconsequentlivercanceristhe
HepatitisBvaccine.Itistypicallyadministeredinaseriesofshots,withthefirstdosefrequentlygivenatbirt
horintheearlyyearsoflife.

PeoplecanprotectthemselvesfromHPVandHepatitisBandlowertheirchanceofcontractingrelatedca
ncersbygettingvaccinatedagainsttheseviruses.It'scrucialtorememberthateventhoughthesevaccin
ationsareverysuccessful,notallcancerscanbecompletelypreventedbythem.Consequently,itisstillcr
ucialtofollowothercancerpreventionguidelines,likegettingregularscreeningsandleadingahealthylif
estyle.

Regardingspecificvaccinationschedulesandrecommendationsbasedonindividualcircumstancesa
ndriskfactors,itisadvisedtoseekadvicefromhealthcareprofessionalsorconsultofficialguidelines.

Early detection and screening

Cancer can be prevented and managed more effectively with early screening and detection. Early cancer detection increases the likelihood of a successful recovery and improves treatment outcomes.

Cancer or precancerous conditions can be detected early on with the use of routine screenings, such as mammograms for breast cancer, Pap tests for cervical cancer, and colonoscopies for colorectal cancer. These examinations look for anomalies or alterations in the body that might point to the existence of cancer or higher chance of getting it.

Timely intervention, such as surgery, radiation therapy, chemotherapy, or targeted therapies, is made possible by early detection. Early detection of cancer often occurs when the disease is more localized, improving treatment options and possibly even curing it.

In addition to screenings, it's critical to recognize possible cancer signs and symptoms and to report any unexpected changes to a healthcare provider right away. Unexpected lumps or growths, persistent fatigue, changes in skin tone, persistent pain, and changes in bowel or bladder habits are some common warning signs.

Reducing the risk of cancer also requires prevention. The risk of developing some types of cancer can be decreased by leading a healthy lifestyle that includes regular exercise, a balanced diet, abstaining from tobacco and excessive alcohol use, and wearing sunscreen to protect oneself from the sun.

It is imperative to acknowledge that although early detection and screening are crucial instruments in the fight against cancer, they cannot ensure the total avoidance or eradication of the disease. Thus, it is crucial to continue taking a proactive approach to general health, which includes routine check-ups and conversations regarding personal risk factors and recommended screenings with medical professionals.

ImportanceofEarlyDetection
Themanagementandpreventionofcancerdependheavilyonearlydetection.Earlycancerdetectionim
provespatientoutcomesoverallanddramaticallyraisesthelikelihoodofasuccessfulcourseoftherapy.
Earlydetectioniscrucialforcancerpreventionforthefollowingmainreasons:

1.MoreTreatmentOptions:Moretreatmentoptionsarefrequentlyavailablewhencancerisdiscoverede
arlyinlife.Treatmentslikesurgery,radiationtherapy,ortargetedtherapiesaremoreeffectiveonearly-
stagecancersbecausetheyaretypicallysmallerandmorelocalized.Higherchancesofafullrecoveryar
dbetterresultsmayresultfromthis.

2.HigherSurvivalRates:Timelyinterventionmadepossiblebyearlydetectionmayraisesurvivalrates.E
arlydetectionofcancerallowsforprompttreatmenttobeginbeforeitspreadstootherpartsofthebody,po
ssiblyimprovinglong-termsurvival.

3.LessIntenseTreatment:Earlycancerdetectionmayhelppreventorlessentheneedforharsh,time-
consumingtherapies.Early-
stagecancersmaysometimesrequirelessinvasiveproceduresorsmallerdosagesofchemotherapyor
adiationtherapy,whichwouldimprovethepatient'squalityoflifeandlessensideeffects.

4.PreventingAdvancedStageCancer:Earlyidentificationcanaidinhaltingthespreadofcancertomore
advancedphases.Interventionssuchaslifestylemodifications,routinescreenings,orpreventivesurge
rycanbeusedtolowertheriskofcancerdevelopmentorprogressionbyidentifyingprecancerouscondit
onsorearlysignsofcancer.

5.Cost-
Effectiveness:Treatingcanceratanearlierstagecanbelessexpensivethantreatingitwhenithasprogre
ssed.Sinceearly-stagetreatmentsaretypicallylessresource-
intensiveandcomplex,theymayalsobelessexpensiveforpatients,healthcaresystems,andsocietyatl
arge.

Awareness-
buildingregardingcancersymptoms,riskfactors,andthevalueofroutinescreeningsiscrucialinorderto
supportearlydetection.Healthprofessionalsshouldbeconsulted,screeningprotocolsshouldbefollow
ed,andpeopleshouldreportanytroublingsymptomsorchangesintheirhealthassoonastheybecomea
pparent.Preventingandtreatingcancermoresuccessfullyispossiblewhenitisdetectedearlyon,giving
peoplethepowertotakechargeoftheirhealth.

CommonScreeningTests(e.gmammograms,colonoscopies)

Avitalpartofcancerpreventionistheuseofroutinescreeningtestslikecolonoscopiesandmammogram
s.Byidentifyingbreastcancerearlyon,mammogramshelppatientsreceivebettertreatmentoutcomesa
ndenableearlyintervention.Ontheotherhand,colorectalcancerandprecancerouspolypscanberemo
vedduringacolonoscopyinordertodetectthediseaseearlyon.

Cancercanbedetectedearlyon,whenitismoretreatable,withtheuseofroutinemammogramsandcolon
oscopies.Accordingtoage,gender,andpersonalriskfactors,thesetestsareadvised.Therightscreenin
gscheduleforeachindividualshouldbedeterminedbyspeakingwithahealthcareprovider.

Rememberthatscreeningtestsarenotinfallible,eventhoughtheyareimportanttoolsinthefightagainstc
ancer.Nothingcanensurethatascreeningtestwillnotrevealcancer,includingfalsepositivesandfalsen
egatives.Becauseofthis,it'scriticaltocombinescreeningwithothercancerpreventionstrategieslikelea
dingahealthylifestyle,abstainingfromtobaccoandexcessivealcoholuse,andadheringtorecommend
edguidelines.

GuidelinesForRegularCheck-upsAndScreenings
Akeyelementofcancerpreventionisroutinescreeningsandcheck-ups.Herearesomebroadprinciplestothinkabout:

1:Speakwithamedicalprofessional:It'simportanttobuildarapportwithaprimarycarephysicianorother healthcareproviderwhocanhelpyoudeterminewhichtestsandexaminationsareappropriateforyoura ge,gender,andpersonalriskfactors.

2.Beawareofyourfamilyhistory:Knowingwhetherornotyouareatahigherriskofdevelopingaparticular ypeofcancerdependsonyourfamily'shistoryofthedisease.Ifnecessary,yourhealthcareprovidercanu sethisinformationtorecommendparticularscreeningsorgenetictesting.

3.Adheretorecommendedguidelines:Anumberoforganizations,includingtheAmericanCancerSocie ty,offerage-andgender-specificguidelinesforcancerscreenings.Theseguidelinesusuallyincludetestrecommendationsforpe rtinentproceduressuchascolonoscopies,Papsmears,andmammograms.Followingtheserecomme ndationsguaranteespromptdetectionandaction.

4.Recognizeyoursymptoms:Althoughscreeningsarenecessary,youshouldalsokeepaneyeoutforan ystrangesymptomsorphysicalchanges.Seeyourhealthcareproviderrightawayifyousufferfromanyp ersistentsymptoms,suchaslumps,irregularbleeding,changesinbowelhabits,orunexplainedweightlo ss.

5.Keepupahealthylifestyle:Eatingwellandlivingahealthylifestylecanhelplowertheriskofcancer.Toba ccoandexcessivealcoholuseshouldbeavoided,abalanceddietshouldbefollowed,regularexercisesh ouldbedone,andexcessivesunexposureshouldbeavoided.

Keepinmindthatspecificsituationsmaydifferfromthoseingeneral,sofollowyourownjudgment.Whend ecidingwhichscreeningandcheck-upscheduleisbestforyourindividualneeds,itisalwaysbesttospeakwithahealthcareprofessional.

CancerRiskAssessmentAndGeneticTesting

Genetictestingandcancerriskassessmentcanbeveryhelpfulinpreventingcancer.Withtheaidoftheset
ools,peoplecanbetterunderstandtheirindividualriskfactorsforacquiringparticularcancertypes,enabl
ingthemtotakepreventativeactionoridentifycancerearlyon.

Todetermineaperson'sriskofdevelopingcancer,anumberoffactorsareassessed,includinglifestylech
oices,environmentalexposures,andfamilyhistory.Thosewhomightbenefitfromfurtherscreeningorpr
eventivemeasurescanbeidentifiedwiththeaidofthisassessment.

Anindividual'sgeneticsusceptibilitytoparticularcancertypescanbeusefullydeterminedthroughgenet
ictesting,particularlyforinheritedgenemutationslikeBRCA1andBRCA2.Thisinformationcandirecttai
oredpreventativemeasures,likeheightenedmonitoringorrisk-minimizingprocedures.

Genetictestingandcancerriskassessmenthelpmedicalprofessionalscustomizepreventivestrategie
sandinterventionsbyidentifyingpeoplewhoaremorelikelytodevelopthedisease.Thiscouldinvolveref
erralstospecializedclinicsorprograms,lifestylechanges,chemoprevention,ormorefrequentscreenin
gs.

Rememberthatalthoughgenetictestingandcancerriskassessmentcanofferinsightfulinformation,the
ycannotensurethatcancerwillnotdevelopornot.Theyareinstrumentstosupportanddirectpreventive
measures.Itisessentialtospeakwithmedicalexpertswhospecializeincancergeneticsinordertocompr
ehendthesignificanceoftestfindingsandcreateapersonalizedpreventivestrategy.

Understandingpersonalriskfactors

Whenitcomestoearlydetectionandcancerprevention,itisessentialtounderstandone'sownriskfactors.Individualswithcertaintraitsorhabitsmaybemoresusceptibletocancer.Theseareknownaspersonalrskfactors.Itispossibleforpeopletolowertheirriskofdevelopingcancerbybeingproactiveandrecognizingtheseriskfactors.

Hereareafewtypicalindividualcancerriskfactors:

1.Age:Aspeopleage,theyaremorelikelytodevelopcancer.Seniorcitizensaremorelikelytodevelopsomecancers,includingcolorectal,prostate,andbreastcancer.

2.Familyhistory:Havingacloserelativewithcancer—aparentorsibling,forexample—canraiseyourriskofgettingsomecancers.Inthesesituations,geneticfactorsmightbeinvolved.

3.Lifestyledecisions:Aperson'schanceofdevelopingcancermayberaisedbycertainlifestyledecisions.Theseincludesmoking,drinkingtoomuchalcohol,eatingpoorly,notexercising,andbeingarounddangerousmaterialslikeasbestosorspecificchemicals.

4.Obesity:Carryingalargeweightorbeingobeseraisestheriskofbreast,colorectal,andpancreaticcancers,amongothercancers.

5.Environmentalfactors:Theriskofacquiringcancercanberaisedbyexposuretocertainenvironmentafactors,suchasradiation,specificchemicals,orpollutants.

Itiscrucialtorememberthataperson'sriskofdevelopingcancerisnotalwaysincreasedbythepresenceofoneormoreriskfactors.Ontheotherhand,thelackofriskfactorsdoesnotensurethatonewillnotdevelopcancer.Individualscan,however,makemoreinformeddecisionsaboutlifestylechoices,screeningoptions,andpreventivemeasuresiftheyareawareoftheirpersonalriskfactors.

Itisadvisedtospeakwithahealthcareprovidertodetermineeachperson'suniqueriskfactors,gooversuitablescreeningtechniques,andcreateacustomizedplanforcancerpreventionandearlydetection.

GeneticTestingAndCounseling
norder to preventand treatcancer,genetictesting and counseling are very important. In genetic testing, a
erson'sDNA is analyzed to find particular gene mutations or alterations that could raise their risk of getting
a particular kind of cancer. People can use this information to lower their risk and make educated decisio
saboutt their healthcare.

Acrucial step in the genetic testing process is genetic counseling. It entails scheduling an appointment wit
a qualified healthcare provider, usually a genetic counselor, who can interpret test results, determine th
person's risk, and offer advice on suitable preventive measures or treatment alternatives. In addition to p
oviding emotional support, genetic counselors also assist clients in comprehending the ramifications of t
st results for their families and themselves.

Genetic testing and counseling can be very beneficial for those with a family history of cancer or specific ge
etic mutations known to increase the risk of cancer. In order to lower their chance of acquiring cancer, it ca
assist in identifying people who might profit from closer monitoring, preventative actions, or even predict
e surgery.

Remember that genetic testing and counseling are intricate procedures requiring serious thought and re
ult interpretation. These are most effectively carried out under the direction of licensed medical professi
nals with cancer and genetics expertise.

PromotingCancerAwarenessAndEducation
norder to effectively combat cancer, it is imperative that cancer awareness and education be promoted.
Byraising awareness of cancer among the general public, we can enable people to take preventative, earl
detection, and management actions.

preading accurate and current knowledge about the causes, risk factors, and symptoms of different typ
s of cancer is one way to raise awareness of the disease. Public service announcements, social media, c
mmunity events, and partnerships with healthcare organizations are just a few of the places these camp
igns can be carried out.

Moreover, educating people about the value of routine screenings and early detection can have a big imp
ct on cancer outcomes. Encouraging people to have the recommended screenings, like colonoscopies
Papsmears, and mammograms, can help detect cancer early on, when treatment is frequently more effe
tive.

One more crucial component of raising awareness and educating people about cancer is encouraging he
lthy lifestyle choices. Some cancers can be prevented by educating people about the advantages of eati
g a balanced diet, exercising frequently, abstaining from tobacco and excessive alcohol use, and shieldi
g oneself from UV radiation.

Itisalsoessentialtoofferresourcesandsupporttocancerpatients,survivors,andtheirfamilies.Informat
onregardingavailablecounselingservices,supportgroups,treatmentoptions,andfinancialaidprogra
mscanallfallunderthiscategory.

Allthingsconsidered,wecanempowerpeopletomakeknowledgeabledecisionsabouttheirhealth,enc
ourageearlydetection,andultimatelylessenthetollthatcancertakesonbothindividualsandsocietyatla
rgebyraisingawarenessofthediseaseandprovidingeducationaboutit.

ImportanceOfCancerEducation

InordertoincreaseawareΩ... encourageprevention,andenhanceoutcomesforthoseimpactedbyca ncer,cancereducationisessential.Thefollowingaresomemainjustificationsforthesignificanceofcanc ereducation:

1.Earlydetection:Peoplewhoreceivecancereducationarebetterabletocomprehendthesignificanceo froutinescreeningsandtheidentificationofearlywarningindicators.Educationcanresultinpromptdiag nosisandpossiblybettertreatmentoutcomesbyencouragingearlydetection.

2.Prevention:Cancereducationoffersguidanceonhealthyeatinghabits,regularexercise,abstainingfr omtobaccoandexcessivealcoholuse,andusingsunscreenprecautions.Educationcanhelplowertheri skofacquiringsometypesofcancerbyencouraginghealthybehaviors.

3.Empowerment:Byprovidinginformationaboutthevariousformsofcancer,availabletreatments,and supportsystems,cancereducationempowerspeople.Withthisknowledge,peoplecanactivelyparticip ateintheirowncare,makeeducateddecisionsregardingtheirhealth,andcollaboratewithhealthcarepro fessionalsondecisions.

4.Supportforcaregivers:Informationandtoolsareprovidedtocaregiversaspartofcancereducationpro gramstohelpthemmanagesideeffectsoftreatment,betterunderstandtheillness,andofferemotionalsu pport.Inordertoguaranteethehealthofpatientsandtheircaregivers,thissupportisessential.

5.Advocacyandpolicyreform:Cancereducationcanserveasacatalystforlobbyingonbehalfoflawsthat advanceequitableaccesstohealthcare,high-qualitycancertreatment,andresearch.Educationhasthepowertopositivelyinfluencefundingandpolic yrelatedtocancerbyenergizingcommunitiesandincreasingawareness.

Allthingsconsidered,cancereducationisessentialforempoweringpeople,encouragingprevention,an denhancingresultsinthebattleagainstthedisease.

SpreadingAwarenessInCommunities
Toencourageearlydetection,prevention,andsupportforthoseimpactedbythedisease,itisimperative
oraisecommunityawarenessofcancer.Inordertoincreasecommunityawarenessofcancer,considert
hefollowingpracticalstrategies:

1.Educationinitiatives:Planinitiativesthatofferpreciseandcurrentinformationonthevariousformsofca
ncer,riskfactors,symptoms,andavailablescreeningtechniques.Webinars,workshops,seminars,an
thedistributionofeducationalmaterialsinpublicareasaresomeofthemethodsthatthesecampaignsca
ntake.

2.Partnershipwithmedicalprofessionals:Arrangehealthfairs,freescreenings,andawarenesscampa
gnsinconjunctionwithneighborhoodclinics,hospitals,andmedicalprofessionals.Inadditiontogivinga
ccesstoresourcesandexpertise,thispartnershipmayhelpreachawideraudience.

3.Involvelocalcelebrities,influencers,andleadersinthecommunity:Theseindividualscanaidinamplif
ingthemessageandexpandingitsreachbyprovidingsupport.Theirparticipationcanbolstercredibilitya
ndmotivateneighborstotakeinitiative.

4.Makeuseofdigitalplatforms:Usewebsites,onlineforums,andsocialmediatosharecancer-
relatedresources,personalaccounts,andeducationalcontent.Participateinlivechats,onlinesupport
roups,orinteractiveQ&Asessionstointeractwiththecommunity.

5.Targethigh-
riskgroups:Determinewhichgroupswithinthecommunityareathighrisk,suchasparticularageranges,
acialorethnicbackgrounds,orprofessions,anddesignawarenesscampaignstospeaktotheirparticula
rneedsanddifficulties.Thisfocusedstrategycanaidinraisingengagementandrelevance.

6.Partnershipwithlocalcommunityorganizations:Incorporatecancerawarenessinitiativesintoyouro
ganization'scurrentprogramsoreventsbyformingpartnershipswithneighborhoodchurches,schools,
businesses,andnon-profits.Existingnetworksandresourcescanbeutilizedinthiscollaboration.

7.Encouragecancersurvivorstosharetheirexperiencesandofferemotionalsupporttoothersbyorgani
zingsupportgroupsandsharingsurvivorstories.Thoseimpactedbycancermayfindthesegroupuplifti
ng,supportive,andawaytofeellessstigmatized.

It'scrucialtokeepinmindthatraisingcommunityawarenessofcancerrequirestheuseofevidence-
basedinformation,culturallysensitivestrategies,andclearcommunication.Wecanmakeabigdifferen
einthefightagainstcancerbyempoweringandincludingmembersofthecommunity.

SupportingCancerResearchAndInitiatives

Encouragingresearchandinitiativesrelatedtocancerisessentialforexpandingourknowledgeoftheilln ess,creatingnoveltreatments,andenhancingtheprognosisofcancerpatients.Thefollowingaresomej ustificationsforwhyit'scriticaltosupportcancerresearchandinitiatives:

1.Scientificdevelopments:Researchoncancerleadstodiscoveriesinsciencethatimproveourknowled geofthedisease'smolecularcauses.Thisinformationaidsinthedevelopmentofcreativestrategiesfortr eatment,earlydetection,andpreventionbyresearchers.Wecanhastenthecreationofnoveltreatments andinterventionsbyfundingresearch.

2.Bettertreatmentoptions:Targetedtherapies,immunotherapies,andprecisionmedicinearejustafew ofthetreatmentoptionsthathaveimprovedasaresultofcancerresearch.Wecankeeprefiningcurrentth erapiesandcreatingmoreindividualized,efficientmethodsthatreducesideeffectsandboostsurvivalrat esbyfundingresearch.

3.Earlydetectionandprevention:Researchendeavorsaugmentthecreationofenhancedscreeningpr otocolsanddiagnosticinstruments,permittingpromptidentificationofcancerduringitsmostamenables tages.Furthermore,researchoffersindividualstheabilitytomakeeducatedlifestyledecisionsthatlower theirriskofcancerbyidentifyingriskfactorsandpreventivetechniques.

4.Patient-centeredcare:Researchincancerfocusesonunderstandingthepsychosocialandsupportivecarenee dsofcancerpatientsinadditiontomedicaladvancements.Wecanenhancethegeneralhealthandqualit yoflifeforcancerpatientsreceivingtreatmentbyendorsingprogramsthatputtheneedsofthepatientfirst.

5.Cooperationandknowledgesharing:Fundingprogramsandresearchoncancerpromotescooperati onbetweenscientists,physicians,andorganizations.Thesharingofinformation,resources,andexperti seisencouragedbythiscollaboration,whichproducesmoreeffectiveandsignificantresearchresults.

6.Policychangeandadvocacy:Fundingcancerresearchandinitiativescanserveasacatalystforeffortst oinfluencepoliciesthatprioritizeaccesstohigh-qualitycancercareandresearch,aswellastoraiseawarenessandsecurefundingfortheseefforts.Weh avethepowertosignificantlyimpactthefightagainstcancerbypromotinggreaterfundingforcancerrese arch.

Finally,fundingcancerresearchandinitiativesiscriticaltoexpandingourknowledgeoftheillness,devel opingnewtreatments,encouragingearlydetectionandprevention,improvingpatientcare,encouragin gteamwork,andinfluencinglegislativechanges.Wecanenhancetheprognosisforthoseafflictedwithth isterribleillnessandachievegreatprogressinthefightagainstcancerbyfundingresearch.

Resourcesandsupportforcancerprevention
Therearenumeroustoolsandsourcesofassistanceavailabletopreventcancer.Thefollowingareimportantdirectionstopursue:

1.HealthcareProfessionals:Forindividualizedadviceoncancerprevention,speakwithyourhealthcareprofessional.Theycanprovideyouinformationonscreenings,immunizations(includinghepatitisBandHPV),andlifestylechangesbasedonyourindividualriskfactors.

2.CancerOrganizations:AwealthofinformationaboutcancerpreventionisavailablefromorganizationssuchastheNationalCancerInstitute,WorldHealthOrganization,andAmericanCancerSociety.Theirwebsitesincludeinformationondifferentcancertypes,riskfactors,andpreventiontechniques,alongwithguidelinesandeducationalmaterials.

3.CommunityInitiatives:Numerouslocalitiesprovidecampaignsandprogramsaimedatpreventingcancer.Supportgroups,awarenesscampaigns,andinstructionalworkshopsareafewexamples.Tolearnabouttheprogramsthatareofferedinyourarea,contactthehealthdepartments,communitycenters,orhospitalsnearby.

4.OnlineResources:Therearealotoftrustworthywebsitesthatofferaccurateinformationaboutcancerprevention.YoucanevaluateyourriskandchoosepreventativestrategieswiththehelpofwebsitessuchasWebMD,MayoClinic,andCancer.gov,whichprovidearticles,guidelines,andtools.

5.SupportGroups:Becomingamemberofasupportgroupforcancersurvivorsorpreventioncanofferinsightfuladviceandencouragement.Theseforumsoftenprovideameansofexchangingexperiences,pickinguptipsfromothers,andgettingaccesstomorepreventativeresources.

6.HealthInsurance:Findoutwhatpreventiveservicesarecoveredbyyourhealthinsurancebycontactingyourprovider.Cancerscreeningsandvaccinationsarenowmorewidelyavailableandreasonablypricedsincemanyinsuranceplanscoverthem.

7.WorkplaceWellnessInitiatives:Afewcompaniesprovidecancerprevention-focusedwellnessinitiatives.Theseinitiativescouldinvolvehealthscreenings,educationalsessions,andrewardsforembracinghealthylifestylechoices.

Recallthatwhenmakingdecisionsregardingcancerprevention,it'scriticaltospeakwithhealthcareprofessionalsandrelyoninformationbasedonevidence.Youcanloweryourriskofdevelopingcancerbyusingthesetoolsandsupportnetworks.

AccessingReliableInformationAndResources
Whenitcomestocancer,itisessentialtohaveaccesstotrustworthyresourcesandinformation.Youcan
makesureyouaregettingreliableinformationbydoingthefollowingsteps:

.Reputablegroups:ConsulttrustworthygroupsliketheWorldHealthOrganization,NationalCancerIn
titute,AmericanCancerSociety,andotherprominentcanceradvocacyandresearchorganizationsfori
formation.Thesegroupsofferinformationbasedonfactsandhaveatrackrecordofreliability.

.Healthcareexperts:Speakwithmedicalexpertslikenurses,primarycaredoctors,andoncologists.Ina
ditiontodirectingyoutotrustworthyresources,theycanofferpreciseandcustomizedinformationbase
onyouruniquecircumstances.

.Internetsources:Usecautionandconfirmthereliabilityofthewebsiteorsourcewhenrelyingoninforma
onfoundonline.Websiteswiththeextensions.gov,.edu,or.orgaremorelikelytohavetrustworthyinfor
ation.Checktheinformationiscurrentandsupportedbyevidencebylookinguppreferences,authorcre
entials,andpublicationdates.

.Supportgroups:Accesstoonlinecommunitiesandsupportgroupsforcancerpatientscanofferinsightf
linformationandhelpfulresources.Butbecarefulwhatyoushare,anddoublechecktheinformationwith
eliablesources.

.ClinicalTrials:SeeyourhealthcareproviderorcheckoutreliablewebsitessuchasClinicalTrials.govify
uwouldliketotakepartinaclinicaltrial.Thesewebsitesofferdetailsaboutcurrenttrials,prerequisites,a
dwaystogetintouchwiththeprovidersofadditionalinformation.

.Locallibrariescanprovidetrustworthyinformationoncancerbecausetheyfrequentlyhaveaccessto
edicaldatabasesandotherresources.Tolocatereliablebooks,journals,andotherresources,youcan
ethelpfromlibrarians.

salways,it'scrucialtoassessmaterialcriticallyandseekoutindividualizedguidancefrommedicalprof
ssionals.

upportiveorganizationsAndservices
ancersurvivorsandtheirfamiliescanfindassistancefromawiderangeoforganizationsandservices.T
giveafewinstances:

.AmericanCancerSociety(ACS):TheACSprovidesacomprehensiverangeofservices,suchasacce
stotreatmentoptions,supportgroups,andinformationresources.Additionally,theysupportcancerpat
entsfinanciallyandwithtransportationandhousing.

2.CancerSupportCommunity:Thisgrouphelpspeoplewithcancerandtheirlovedonesbyofferingfree supportgroups,educationalworkshops,andcounseling.Inadditiontoprovidingonlineassistance,they avelocalchaptersalloverthecountry.

3.NationalCancerInstitute(NCI):Aninformationalwebsiteaboutcancertreatmentoptions,clinicaltria s,supportivecare,andothercancer-
relatedtopics,NCIisafederalagencythatcarriesoutcancerresearch.Patients,caregivers,andhealthc areprofessionalscanaccessawealthofresourcesontheirwebsite.

4.TheLivestrongFoundation:Forcancerpatients,theLivestrongFoundationprovidesfinancialsuppo ,counseling,andone-on-oneguidance.Forcaregiversandsurvivorsalike,theyofferresources.

5.CancerCare:Supportgroups,financialaid,educationalworkshops,andfreeprofessionalcounselin areallofferedtocancerpatientsbyCancerCare.Theirservicesareavailablenotonlyonlineandoverthe hone,butalsoinperson.

6.HospiceandPalliativeCareOrganizations:Themissionofthesegroupsistosupportandcomfortpatie ntswithadvancedcancerandtheirfamilies.Theyprovidehelpwithend-of-
lifecaredecisions,painmanagement,andemotionalsupport.

7.LocalSupportGroups:Therearenumerouslocalsupportgroupsinmanycommunitiesthatarededica edtohelpingcancerpatientsandsurvivors.Thesecommunitiesofferasecuresettingforexchangingsto ies,offeringconsolation,anddispensingcounsel.

Rememberthatdependingonwhereyoulive,theseorganizations'andservices'accessibilitymaychan ge.Youcanfindmorelocalresourcesandsupportnetworksbyspeakingwithsocialworkers,healthcare rofessionals,orcancertreatmentfacilities.

EngagingInSupportiveNetworkAndCommunities

Participatingincommunitiesandnetworksofsupportcanbeextremelybeneficialforpeopledealingwith arangeofissues,includingcancer-relatedissues.Participatingincommunitiesandnetworksthatprovidesupportiscrucialforthefollowingreasons:

1.Emotionalsupport:Communitiesandsupportivenetworksofferaforumforpeopletointeractwithotherswhohavegonethroughcomparableexperiences.Itcanbereassuring,validating,andafeelingofcommunitytosharefeelings,fears,andworrieswithotherswhogetit.Peoplewhoreceivethisemotionalsupportarebetterabletomanagethepsychologicaleffectsofcancerandexperiencelessfeelingsofloneliness.

2.Resourcesandinformation:Communitiesandsupportivenetworksfrequentlyprovideaccesstoimportantcancer-relatedresources,information,andeducationalmaterials.Toassistpeopleinnavigatingthechallengesofcancerdiagnosis,treatment,andsurvivorship,memberscanexchangetheirexpertise,personalstories,andusefuladvice.Peoplemaybebetterequippedtomakedecisionsabouttheircareasaresultofthisinformationsharing.

3.Realisticsupport:Communitiesandsupportnetworkscanalsoofferrealisticsupportintheformofmealdelivery,transportation,orassistancewitheverydayduties.Withthehelpofthesedeedsofcompassion,peoplecanfocusontheirwell-beingandlessenthestressofreceivingcancertreatment.

4.Empowermentandadvocacy:Participatingincommunitiesandnetworksofsupportcanprovidepeoplethechancetotakeontheroleofadvocatesforboththemselvesandotherpeople.Peoplecaninfluencefavorablechangesincancer-relatedlegislation,fundingforresearch,andaccesstohigh-qualitycarebysharingtheirexperiences,spreadingawareness,andtakingpartinadvocacycampaigns.

5.Inspirationandhope:Speakingwithpeoplewhohavesurmountedcomparableobstaclescanprovideinspirationandhope.Thosefacingtheirownstrugglescanfindinspirationandhopefromseeingotherswhohavesuccessfullynavigatedtheircancerjourney.

Allthingsconsidered,beingapartofsupportivecommunitiesandnetworkscanofferasenseofhope,advocacyopportunities,practicalhelp,emotionalsupport,andaccesstoresourcesandinformation.TheserelationshipscanhaveasubstantialimpactonthehealthandThestandardoflivingforthoseimpactedbycancer.

Conclusion

Inconclusion,avarietyoffactors,includingasgenetics,environmentalexposures,lifestyledecisions,ar
dspecificinfections,cancontributetothedevelopmentofcancer.Ontheotherhand,wecantakeactionto
preventcancerandenhancetheprognosisofcancerpatientsthrougheducationandawareness.People
canactivelycontributetotheirownwell-
beingbyrealizingthevalueofearlydetection,forminghealthyhabits,andusingavailableresourcesforsu
pport.

It'scrucialforcancerpatientstokeepinmindthattheyarenottravelingthisjourneyalone.Seekouttheemo
tionalandpracticalsupportoflovedones,supportgroups,andmedicalprofessionals.Remainuptodate
onyourdiagnosis,availableresources,andtreatmentoptions.Alwaysremembertoputself-
carefirstandhaveanoptimisticoutlook.

Eventhoughlivingwithcancercanbedifficult,itiscrucialtomaintainoptimismandfortitude.Concentrate
ontheaspectsofyourtreatmentplan,healthylifestylemaintenance,andseekingoutemotionalsupport
whenrequired.Thesearethethingsyoucancontrol.Keepinmindthatthereisnoone-size-fits-
allstrategyfortreatingcancer;everyperson'sexperienceisdifferent.Haveasolidsupportnetworkarour
dyou,andwhenthingsgettough,youcanrelyonit.

Finally,keepupyouradvocacyforcancerpatients,includingyourself.Tellyourstory,createawareness,
andlendyoursupporttoprogramsthatadvancecancerresearch,betterhealthcareaccess,andimprove
dlegislation.Whenweworktogether,thebattleagainstcancercanbewon.

Staystrong,stayinformed,andknowthatthereishopeandsupportavailabletoyou.